Sergiy Tyupa
Diane Wild

Translating Clinical Trial Outcomes Measures

An overview

SEEd

Via Magenta, 35 – 10128 Torino (Italy)
Tel. +39.011.566.02.58
www.edizioniseed.it – info@edizioniseed.it

First edition October 2016
ISBN 978-88-97419-71-6

Although the information about medication given in this book has been carefully checked, the author and publisher accept no liability for the accuracy of this information. In every individual case the user must check such information by consulting the relevant literature.

Summary

Introduction

The purpose of this book is to provide a general overview of the translation and cultural adaptation process of clinical research survey instruments with a focus on the linguistic aspects of the process. Survey instruments here refer to any text, printed or electronic, prepared in order to collect information in a clinical research setting. This broad definition covers patient-reported, clinician-reported, and caregiver-reported outcomes measures, as well as patient diaries, indexes, scales, symptom checklists, etc. The target audience includes translation agencies that specialize in the translation of clinical research survey instruments, contract research organizations and their respective translation departments, regulators, industry, and academia.

The book is made up of two parts. The first part offers a brief introduction to selected linguistic aspects of translation. Its purpose is twofold: firstly, to provide definitions of key linguistic concepts that will be used in the following chapters, and secondly, to set a tentative theoretical framework for the translation and cultural adaptation process. The second part describes the main steps used in the translation process. It relies heavily on the *"Principles of Good Practice for the Translation and Cultural Adaptation Process for Patient-Reported Outcomes (PRO) Measures"* [Wild, 2005]. The original Principles of Good Practice (PGP) identified ten steps:

1. Preparation;
2. Forward Translation;
3. Reconciliation;
4. Back Translation;
5. Back Translation Review;

6. Harmonization;
7. Cognitive Debriefing;
8. Review of Cognitive Debriefing Results and Finalization;
9. Proofreading;
10. Final Report.

These steps have been rearranged and modified in order to optimize the presentation of material and also to reflect the most recent trends and developments in the area of translation and cultural adaptation. Since the book focuses almost exclusively on the linguistic aspects of translation, the irrelevant procedures have been removed from the discussion, and new, more relevant ones, have been added. Thus, the Preparation step now includes a new process that has recently received growing attention in Clinical Outcomes Assessment (COA) development and linguistic validation community, namely, Translatability Assessment. Forward Translation and Reconciliation are described in one chapter since the two steps are closely interconnected and interdependent. For the same reason, Back Translation, Back Translation Review and Harmonization are presented in one chapter. The Proofreading step has been extended to include Check, Revision and Review, in line with the new ISO 17100:2015 standards for translation services. The preparation of the Final Report has not been included in the discussion as it is not relevant for the description of linguistic aspects.

The discussion of each step includes the definition of its most important components, a list of key professionals involved in implementing the step, a detailed critical description of the processes involved in the implementation of the step, as well as a brief overview of areas where more research is needed. The latter component was added because we felt that the translation and cultural adaptation process should be based on sound empirical evidence drawn both from daily practice of language professionals as well as high quality research initiatives.

The final chapter covers the translation of electronic versions of clinical research survey instruments, with a brief discussion of the necessary modifications of each step in order to meet the needs of an electronic instrument translation.

SECTION I

Linguistic Aspects of Translation

Key terms and definitions

CONCEPT

Concept is one of the key terms used in literature on clinical research survey instruments, especially in publications on the translation and cultural adaptation process. In a more specific field of PRO instruments, the Food and Drugs Administration (FDA) defines a concept as "the *thing* being measured, such as a symptom or group of symptoms, effects on a particular function or group of functions, or a group of symptoms or functions shown to measure the severity of a health condition" [FDA, 2009]. There is an important difference in how this term is understood in linguistics.

In the studies of language and in cognitive science in general a *concept* is viewed as a dynamic mental knowledge structure that relates to some entity (*referent*) in the experienced world. The entity that the concept relates to could be a material object, an event, a situation, an experience, an emotion, an attitude, a relation, and, importantly, a schematic generalization thereof. These generalized concepts help humans to structure reality into relevant categories, referred to as *conceptual categories* [Dirven, 2004]. Some, but certainly not all concepts and conceptual categories give rise to *linguistic categories*, i.e. words and linguistic structures that represent these concepts and conceptual categories. A

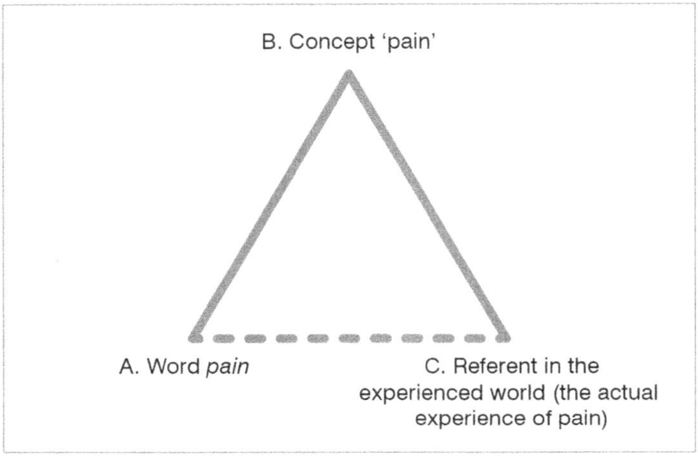

Figure 1. *Semiotic triangle. Modified from [Ogden, 1923]*

simplified illustration for the relations between words, concepts, and referents in the experienced world is known as a *semiotic triangle* and was introduced by Ogden and Richards as far back as 1923 [Ogden, 1923]. Its modified version is presented in Figure 1 below, with the concept of 'pain' as an example.

A solid line from A to B indicates that there is a direct link between the form of the word *pain* in English and the concept of 'pain' in the mind of an English-speaker. In other words, the word *pain* is a point of access to the concept of 'pain' and the related conceptual categories, as there is evidence to believe that a word evokes not individual concepts, but complex structures thereof. A solid line between B and C indicates that there is equally a direct link between the concept of 'pain' and the actual experience of pain. In other words, when a person experiences pain she thinks of pain, which is self-evident. However, there is no direct link between the word and the thing or referent for which it stands, so the line between A and C is interrupted.

If we go back to the FDA definition of *concept,* where it is equated with a *thing,* it becomes clear now that a *concept* is mixed up with a *referent*, i.e. the thing in the experienced world that the concept represents. Consequently, when the FDA guidance says that the "concepts measured by PRO instruments that are most often used in support of labelling claims refer to a patient's symptoms, signs, or an aspect of functioning directly related to disease status" [FDA, 2009] it is important to realize that PRO instruments and other clinical research survey instruments measure not the symptoms and signs as such, but their conceptual representations in the minds of respondents.

This has equally important consequences for the translation and cultural adaptation process. The basic premise is that the conceptual categories that represent symptoms, signs, and aspects of functioning are adequately similar in the minds of speakers of different languages. If we did not agree on this premise, this would render international comparison of data impossible. From a common sense perspective, it would also be odd to expect that a speaker of Japanese experiences, for example, increased body temperature differently from a speaker of Spanish. The difference lies in the representation of conceptual categories through linguistic categories, and the main task of the translation and cultural adaptation process is to find such linguistic categories in the target language that give access to conceptual categories that are sufficiently close to the concepts evoked in the source language.

A vivid example is the translation of word forms that represent a complex conceptual category of 'pain' in English. Clinical research survey instruments often use two distinct word forms, namely *pain* and *ache*, to refer to different aspects of the conceptual category of 'pain' that investigators are interested in. The English language has developed two individual words that stand for these aspects, whereas in many other languages there are no corresponding single words for 'ache' and for 'pain'[1]. The solution is to provide a descriptive translation, usually with the help of words that stand for characteristics of pain (e.g. *sharp, dull,*

---

[1] Just like with many other synonyms in the English language, *ache* originated from Old English and can be traced back to the 9th century, whereas *pain* was borrowed from Old French in late 13th century (Chambers Dictionary of Etymology 2008).

prolonged, acute, etc.), that would evoke the same concepts in the target language that the original English words *ache* and *pain*. Therefore, when papers on the translation and cultural adaptation process claim that there may be an absence of some concepts in target languages, it actually may mean that there are no established word forms to represent these concepts, but it does not mean that an adequate translation cannot be found, as the relevant concepts can be accessed with the help of more elaborated and detailed linguistic expressions.

MEANING

Meaning is another key notion for the translation and cultural adaptation of clinical research survey instruments. From a very simplified perspective, it can be said that meaning is identical to a concept [Dirven, 2004]. However, such a definition is not sufficient for the discussion of complex phenomena involved in the translation process. Meaning is studied by a dedicated discipline of semantics, but it is also the object of interest in philosophy, logic, psychology, semiotics. The challenge is to find a proper theoretical framework that would be relevant for this discussion, and at the same time would be clear and concise enough to eliminate the need for an extensive introduction. We believe that cognitive linguistics meets these criteria. Cognitive linguistics is currently one of the most influential, albeit loosely structured [Geeraerts, 2010], approaches to the study of language, which has recognised the problem of meaning as central for linguistic research. The following summary will be largely based on a work by Langacker [Langacker, 2008], one of the leading figures in cognitive linguistics.

One of the most important aspects of meaning is its dynamic nature. Meanings are not entirely fixed and predetermined, as could be misleadingly suggested by dictionary definitions. Instead, the speaker and the hearer[2] actively negotiate meanings, depending on the circumstances of the situation, the physical environment, the social and cultural context, their linguistic abilities, the communication channel, and many other factors. Therefore, meaning should be identified not with concepts, but with conceptualization:

> «Conceptualization is broadly defined to encompass any facet of mental experience. It is understood as subsuming 1) both novel and established conceptions; 2) not just "intellectual" notions, but sensory, motor, and emotive experience as well; 3) apprehension of the physical, linguistic, social, and cultural context; and 4) conceptions that develop and unfold through processing time (rather than being simultaneously manifested)» [Langacker, 2008].

This does not mean, however, that in every speech situation meanings are negotiated "from scratch". Instead, interlocutors have preconceptions of the meanings of words. These preconceptions develop through communicative interactions that language users have in their speech community. It can be safely claimed that most of the misunderstandings of source texts that appear during the translation process can be explained by the fact that translators lack experience with such 'communicative interactions' in the source language community, and not by, for example, lack of good dictionaries.

The dynamic nature of conceptualization can be illustrated with the following example. PRO questionnaires with multiple response options commonly use the verb *choose* in the instructions on filling in questionnaires, as in "Please choose one response option per each question". The conceptualization of the word *choose* as an action that needs to be performed by the respondent will be different depending on the mode of administration of the questionnaire, on the type of the instrument (printed or

[2] 'Speaker' and 'hearer' are used here as technical terms that refer to both spoken and written communication. A speaker, for example, could be the developer of a clinical research survey instrument, and the hearer – the translator who works on its translation.

Context	Conceptualization of choose
A questionnaire administered by a clinician, with questions read to the respondent	«Verbally tell the number of the response options to the clinician»
A printed questionnaire completed by a respondent	«Place some visible mark next to the response option»
An electronic questionnaire completed by a respondent	«Click the response options that I choose»
An IVRS questionnaire completed by a respondent during a phone call	«Press the number of the response option on the telephone keyboard»

Table I. *Alternative conceptualizations of 'choose'*

electronic), and on many other "physical, linguistic, social, and cultural" aspects of context referred to in the quote above. Table I summarizes alternative conceptualizations of *choose* depending on the context of a speech situation.

It is important to mention that the translation of the verb *choose* may be different depending on the context, therefore, without the knowledge of the broad context of a given questionnaire, a translator may fail to choose the most appropriate term for *choose* in the target language. For example, if the translator is not aware that the questionnaire will be administered with children, he or she may use the verb *choose* in an official form of address (e.g. in the second person plural imperative form in the case of Ukrainian), which is not suitable when addressing children.

Another essential aspect of linguistic meaning, relevant for the translation process, is the relation between the total body of knowledge that we have about a certain entity and the meaning of the word or words that represent this entity in our conceptual system. Traditionally, the meaning of individual words (the lexical meaning) is described through a limited set of descriptive statements, similar to definitions that we find in dictionaries. Hence, this approach is known as the *dictionary* view of the lexical meaning, where all the knowledge that speakers have about a certain entity is not considered necessary for describing the meaning of the lexical items that stand for this entity. Cognitive linguistics takes a different approach, known as *encyclopaedic semantics*. According to this approach, a "lexical meaning resides in a particular way of accessing an open-ended body of knowledge pertaining to a certain type of entity" [Langacker, 2008]. The difference between these two approaches can be best explained with the help of an example.

It is not uncommon for instructions of clinical research survey instruments to start with a personal pronoun *we,* as in "We are interested in learning how you have been doing over the past couple of days". According to the dictionary view, the lexical item *we* here means "reference to a group including the speaker and at least one other person"[3]. If the instrument is self-administered, there are actually no 'speakers' that respondents can link the pronoun *we* with. Consequently, if we take the dictionary view, a respondent can only understand *we* as referring to some unidentified group consisting of at least two persons. However, this is not the intended meaning of the instrument developers, as they expect that the respondent will understand *we* as referring to the study team, or the instrument authors, or investigators, or physicians, etc.

This means that the authors, consciously or not, presuppose that respondents should have some knowledge about clinical research, about the relevant roles of investigators or physicians, about the function of questionnaires, etc. Therefore, as stated above, the pronoun *we* serves as an access point to the total body of knowledge that respondents may (and according to the instrument authors – must) have about clinical researchers that ask questions through structured questionnaires. This means that the dictionary view to meaning is to all intents and purposes rejected by speakers in their actual linguistic practice, and the encyclopaedic understanding of expressions – implicitly expected from hearers.

From a translator's perspective the use of *we* in this context may be problematic. One does not need to be an expert in cogni-

[3] Definition from Cambridge Dictionary (http://dictionary.cambridge.org/dictionary/english/we, accessed on July 17, 2016)

tive linguistics to understand that the use of *we* can be too vague in many languages and cultures, especially those where a research situation with the use of questionnaires is not particularly common. In other words, translators are often restricted not by the absence of lexical expressions (a pronoun or a distinct morpheme to represent the category of the first person plural is present in virtually all languages), but by the absence of relevant knowledge structures that the expressions should give access to.

In sum, meaning can be equated with conceptualization, a dynamic cognitive process of interaction between existing and emerging conceptual categories representing embodied human experience. Lexical meaning is encyclopaedic in nature, in that lexical expressions (words) provide points of access to the open-ended body of knowledge that we have about the entities (referents) represented by words. The immediate significance of this view on meaning for the translation and cultural adaptation is that all participants of any translation project should be given the maximum possible context and information about the instrument that is being translated in order to ensure adequate understanding of the source text.

Selected areas of linguistic research

Modern linguistics offers a variety of research topics that can be extremely useful for the translation and cultural adaptation in particular and for the development of clinical research survey instruments in general. Below we focus on three such fields selected for their immediate relevance to international clinical research and offer a brief summary of each. However, it should be emphasized that this is only a very limited selection from a varied and multifaceted field of linguistic research.

STUDIES OF EMOTIONS IN LANGUAGES

Words that people use to speak about emotions play an extremely important role in clinical research survey instruments, especially in PRO questionnaires, as they are intended to capture signs and symptoms represented through various emotional states, such as anger, fear, anxiety, sadness, etc. Just like in most other aspects of clinical research survey instruments, the success or failure of an instrument measuring certain emotions critically depends the language used. In addition, as linguists working on the study of emotion words argue, "[t]hese questions have to be approached seriously, for the validity of scientific studies of emotional response may depend upon whether the issue of language is addressed in an informed way or by default" [Harkins, 2001].

Linguistics in general and lexical semantics in particular has a lot to offer to researchers to ensure that they make informed decisions about the use of emotion words.

The challenge, however, is to identify the literature, as publications on emotion words are scattered in academic journals, in edited volumes (e.g. [Harkins, 2001]), and in monographs (e.g. [Kövecses, 1986], [Dewaele, 2010], [Dziwirek, 2010]). Besides, linguists usually focus on a particular emotion or a group of emotions, for instance, concepts of anger in Chinese [Kornacki, 2001], so a certain synthesis from the available works would be necessary in order to make them applicable to clinical research. One of the ways to tackle these difficulties would be to invite professional linguists[4] to instrument development teams and to translation and cultural adaptation teams.

In sum, the value of linguistic research into emotion words and concepts cannot be overstressed. One of the first steps in acknowledging the importance of language for clinical research would be to recognize the fact that a lot of decisions are made through the prism of English, which inevitably introduces bias into research. Researchers should keep in mind that "we cannot treat English emotion words such as *anger* as neutral, self-explanatory, and culture-independent terms by means of which human emotional experience in all cultures can be validly and meaningfully described" [Harkins, 2001]. Naturally, this applies not only to emotion words but to the English lexicon in general.

CORPUS STUDIES

Corpus linguistics is a cover term to refer to various research endeavours based on large digital linguistic databases known as

[4] The term *linguist* is used here to refer to academics pursuing research in linguistics, and not to language services professionals, such as translators and editors, as this term is sometimes understood in clinical research publications.

corpora. For example, the British National Corpus (www.natcorp.ox.ac.uk/) contains about 100 million words of both written (about 90% of the corpus) and spoken language. Similar corpora exist or are being developed for many other languages. Besides, linguists build their own corpora from different texts depending on specific purposes of their research. The obvious advantage of corpus linguistics is that language is studied on the basis of numerous real-life samples of language use, rather than isolated examples hand-picked by linguists. The results of corpus-based linguistic research could be used in the translation and cultural adaptation process, however, with the need to tackle the same challenges described in section "Studies of emotions in languages". We offer a summary of one of the corpus-based research papers as an illustration of the possible added value that corpus linguistics may bring into clinical research and the translation process.

The study in question [Glynn, 2010] is based on a sample of 650 occurrences of the word *bother* in British and American English[5]. The samples were randomly selected from on-line blogs, so they represent language as used by lay speakers – similarly to how items for survey instruments are being generated based on input from focus groups made up of representatives of the target population. The samples were analysed along a number of formal and semantic features, each representing an independent variable. The most subjective variables were annotated independently by two linguists. Cohen's Kappa was used to establish the degree of inter-coder agreement. For each of the four subjective variables Cohen's Kappa was approaching 1, which is considered perfect agreement. Correspondence Analysis was used to identify three basic senses of the word *bother.* Two of the sense clusters were verified with the help of Logistic Regression Analysis.

---

5 The word *bother* and associated concepts prove to be some of the most difficult in translation and cultural adaptation of clinical research survey instruments, which provides additional rationale for choosing Glynn's research as an illustration of corpus studies.

Senses	Pain	Annoyance	Hassle
Affect	The experiencer feels hurt by physical pain through emotional pain to general psychological stress	The experiencer feels imposed upon or prevented from doing what he or she wishes to do	The experiencer feels put out by the need to do something that involves the use of energy
Agent	Friends and family and other known individuals, states and abstract states of affairs	People, especially people that the experiencer does not personally know	Events, basically 'having to do things'

Table II. *Corpus-based senses of bother [Glynn, 2010]*

As the result of the conducted analyses it was possible to single out three distinct senses of *bother* that come not from dictionary definitions or the subjective interpretation of a linguist, but from real-world usage-based data that was subjected to "operationalised, verified, and statistically confirmed treatment" [Glynn, 2010]. These three senses are presented in Table II. *Affect* stands for the emotions and feelings involved, *Agent* refers to an entity that brings about a given sense of *bother*. *Experiencer* means the person who experiences a state described by one of the senses of *bother*.

The study presented above belongs to some of the most sophisticated types of corpus-based research. However, one does not need to have special training in linguistics in order to be able to use some of the basic features of electronic open-access corpora that still will be helpful in making informed decisions about language issues. For example, it is possible to check the frequency of linguistic expressions in the corpus, the contexts in which they are used, the types of texts where they appear, etc. Similar correspondence searches can be done for expressions that are deemed equivalent in the target languages. Finally, the use of language corpora for the development of new instruments seems not only possible, but also necessary.

STUDIES OF METAPHOR

Metaphor is commonly understood as a figure of speech which refers to one entity as being the same as another entity. One of the most famous metaphors is Shakespeare's "All world's a stage", but the fact is that metaphor is much more ubiquitous in language and can be found in areas very distant from literature. Take, for example, the phrase "Investigators are blinded to the results of the experiment". Here, *blinded* is used in a figurative, metaphoric sense, and it is hard to imagine that someone would see a direct, non-figurative meaning of *blind* here. However, the usage of *blind* as a clinical research term could be traced back to the first use of this word by some researcher who used language creatively to describe a situation when some information is kept hidden from investigators/patients[6]. Modern linguistics goes even further than this and claims that metaphoric thinking belongs to some of the basic features of our cognition.

This school of thought is known as the conceptual theory of metaphor [Lakoff, 1980] [Lakoff, 1987]. It distinguishes novel metaphors, usually found in literary works or in some original writing or speech, from conventionalized metaphors that normally are not recognized as metaphors by language users. Some novel metaphors get conventionalized, as in the example of *blinded* above. What is important for our discussion is that "certain metaphors are conventionalized again and again across languages, while others are not" [Croft, 2004]. Lakoff and his colleagues believe that this can be explained by the significance of a given metaphor in human cognitive system, which in turn is based on embodied human experience. By *experience* we mean such fundamental aspects as the experience of three-dimensional space, time, temperature, exertion of force, etc., as well as experiences unique to a certain cultural group.

Therefore, in the most simplified terms a conceptual metaphor is the understanding of something that is not known to us

6 To the best of our knowledge, no such study has been conducted so far.

(*target domain*) in terms of something that is known (*source domain*). Another way of explaining the difference between source and target domains would be presenting them as a dichotomy of concrete (source domain) versus abstract (target domain). Thus, anger as an abstract feeling is often expressed with the help of an underlying conceptual metaphor ANGER IS HEAT OF A FLUID IN A CONTAINER[7] [Lakoff, 1987], as physical containers containing hot liquids are common in human life and belong to basic physical experience of the world. This conceptual metaphor can be illustrated with the following phrases (all taken from [Lakoff, 1987]):

- She got *all steamed up*;
- Billy's just *blowing off steam*;
- I was *fuming*;
- I was *bursting with anger*;
- I could barely *contain* my rage;
- He *turned his anger inward*;
- When I told him, he just *exploded*;
- We won't tolerate any more of your *outbursts*.

The key question for the discussion of translation and cultural adaptation is therefore how universal conceptual metaphors are, how easily do they translate[8] across cultures. Clinical research survey instruments, especially PRO questionnaires, psychological tests, and other patient-facing materials abundantly use conventionalized metaphors, such as *to be down, mood swings, to be in low spirits, to take what other people say, to find it hard to do something, to feel mixed up,* etc. There is no one-fit-for-all solution for translating metaphors, but at least recognizing the fact that there is a source domain where the conventionalized metaphor comes from could be the key for its proper understanding.

Moreover, conceptual metaphors can be more abstract and manifest themselves not only in proper linguistic expression. For

[7] Source and target domains are usually represented in capital letters.

[8] The verb *translate* itself stems from Latin *trānslātus*, a past participle of *trānsferre* – 'to bring over, carry over'. Here we have a metaphoric extension from a concrete (move objects in space) to a more abstract action.

example, visual analogue scales that offer a 0 (zero) as the worst possible option and 10 as the best possible option rely on one of the most basic conceptual metaphors UP IS BETTER[9]. The question arises then whether it is justified to use scales with the opposite value of anchors. Besides, it has not been convincingly proven that this metaphor is universal across all cultures.

In this section we presented only a few of the many possible areas of linguistic research that are immediately relevant for the translation and cultural adaptation of clinical research survey instruments. However, we believe that even the awareness of such basic linguistic problems will help researchers make more informed decisions.

[9] This metaphor stems, again, from our basic human experience: healthy people are normally erect, whereas ill people usually lie down.

SECTION II

Translation and Cultural Adaptation Process

Preparation

Successful preparation may ensure success at later stages of any complex project, including translation and cultural adaptation. The preparation step involves both linguistic and non-linguistic aspects. The latter include seeking the permission to use and translate the chosen instrument from its developers or copyright holders, as well as selecting teams of translation professionals for respective target languages. These processes will not be discussed here. The linguistic aspects of the preparation step are the following:

- Preparation of source files;
- Concept elaboration;
- Translatability assessment.

The key players involved in this step are: project managers, linguistic consultants, clients, and instrument developers. Project managers are coordinators of a translation project who work for a Language Service Provider (LSP). An LSP can be an in-house translation department of a Contract Research Organization (CRO) or an individual translation agency. Linguistic consultants are professional translators with extensive experience in the translation of clinical research survey instruments. Clients are pharmaceutical companies or other entities that sponsor the translation of the instrument; they may participate in the process directly or through a CRO. Instrument developers are individuals or organizations that developed the respective instrument.

PREPARATION OF SOURCE FILES

The preparation of source files does not comprise only technical issues, such as converting the original instrument into the file format that translators will be working on. More importantly, the source files need to be analyzed from the linguistic perspective before they are split into segments that will be used during the translation workflow. The splitting of the source text into segments is practically inevitable today since the translation of survey instruments is almost never done in the original document format. However, this has to be done very carefully in order to avoid possible problems during the following steps of the translation process.

The source text can be split into segments either manually or automatically. The former approach, currently almost obsolete, is used when the translation is carried out only in simple text editors (such as MS Word). The latter approach comes into play when Computer-Aided Translation (CAT) software tools are used, such as SDL Trados, MemoQ, Memsource, etc. So why is it necessary to analyze the source files first and only then carry out the segmenting or improve the automatic CAT segmentation? The answer lies in the special structure of clinical research survey instruments. Since they are used as measurement tools, there is little plain text (i.e. simple sentence-after-sentence, paragraph-based structure). Instead, survey instruments often contain incomplete question stems, multiple response options, graphic elements, visual analogue scales, illustrations, lists and many other special features. Poor segmenting is likely to cause translation errors or at least increase the amount of time and effort spent during the following translation steps.

Another important aspect to consider while preparing source files is the use of a so-called 'legacy translation'. Legacy translation refers to previous translated versions of an instrument that are used as the basis for producing the translations of an updated instrument. It is natural that clients and developers insist that no changes can be made in the legacy translation, as in most cases the translation has already gone through an expensive linguistic validation process and may have already been used in a research setting. Changing the legacy translation would, in the clients' and developers' opinion, compromise the comparability and validity of data. However, we believe there should always be a possibility to allow translators to introduce changes to the legacy translation. The most important reasons for this are the following:

- Errors. Even the most thorough translation processes cannot guarantee an absolutely error-free translation, not to mention translations that were done many years ago, when there were no or few translation quality assurance tools in place and no standard translation methodology.
- Linguistic changes. These changes may take a radical form of an orthography reform (e.g. in German-speaking countries in 1996), or of slower and less noticeable natural changes in vocabulary, grammar, language users' preferences, acceptable degree of formality, etc.
- Extra-linguistic changes. A lot of instruments, especially those that collect demographic information, refer to referents in the real world, such as medical and educational institutions, names of professions, types of employment, etc. Such referents may change with time, e.g. an institution of a family physician may be introduced in a country where previously there was no family medicine.

It is impossible to foresee all potential segmenting and legacy translation issues since every instrument is unique. The Table III presents only the most common structuring elements of survey instruments and legacy translation features that have to be taken into account when reviewing the source documents prior to segmenting, as well as possible solutions that may help to avoid translation problems.

Source document element	Possible issues	Solutions
Headers and footers	Some text in headers or footers, such as the acronym of an instrument or the names of companies and organizations, is not intended for translation. Other elements, such as the date, the word 'page' etc. have to be translated.	Place the portion of text that has to be translated into a different segment. If this is not possible for technical reasons, clearly mark the text not intended for translation with the help of the respective tag functions in CAT tools.
Incomplete question stems	Clinical research survey instruments often contain questions with an incomplete stem followed by a number of response options. Example: *How often over the past 7 days have you felt...* *a. upset?* *b. tired?* The possible issue is that the choice of an equivalent for a response option depends on the preceding question stem (e.g. some response options may have to be rendered as adjectives, and others as nouns, etc.). This issue is also relevant for Translation Memories (TMs) used by CAT tools: even though a memory may indicate a 100% match, the response option may not be suitable for a new question stem. This is particularly dangerous when such segments are marked as 'perfect match' or 'context match' in CAT tools and are locked by project managers as legacy translation.	Add the question stem in square brackets before each response option and tag it as text not intended for translation. Example: *[How often over the past 7 days have you felt]... tired?* Disable the automatic propagation function or its equivalent in a CAT tool. Avoid locking legacy translation segments in a CAT tool.

Table continues >

> Table continued

Source document element	Possible issues	Solutions
Response options	Even if questions in a PRO instrument are complete, identical response options may need to be changed depending on the question that they refer to. Example: *1. How would you describe your health over the past 7 days?* *a. Excellent* *b. Good* *c. ...* *2. How would you describe your mood over the past 7 days?* *a. Excellent* *b. Good* *c. ...* In many languages, the response options will have to be different as 'health' and 'mood' may be of a different grammatical gender.	Add segments with response options after each question, even if the response options are identical. Disable the automatic propagation function or its equivalent in a CAT tool.

Table III. *Preparation of source documents: issues and solutions*

CONCEPT ELABORATION

Concept elaboration refers to a detailed explanation of terms and concepts used in the source document. A concept elaboration may also include background information on the instrument, the study where it is to be used, the target population, etc. Its primary purpose is to ensure that translators interpret the concepts according to the original intention of the instrument developers. To put it into simple words, concept elaboration helps translators to correctly understand the source document. This immediately implies that whoever prepares the concept elaboration must, in their turn, fully understand the source document items. In most contexts this presupposes direct communication with instrument developers. Overall, there are three main stages in preparing concept elaboration documents:

1. Selecting items and/or concepts that need to be elaborated;
2. Preparing draft definitions;
3. Validating draft definitions with instrument developers.

As will be argued below, we believe that concept elaboration has to be closely connected with translatability assessment. Concept elaboration definitions can be verified and improved during the translatability assessment process. Therefore, this introduces an additional stage:

4. Updating concept elaboration definitions based on translatability assessment results.

Selection of items

There are different approaches to selecting items for concept elaboration. Some LSPs prefer to develop extensive definitions for all items, whereas others select only the most complicated ones. Besides, concept elaboration definitions may explain an item as a whole or just define individual words. Respective decisions are made on the basis of company policies, client preferences, budget constraints, and many other factors. Nevertheless, some general recommendations applicable to most situations can be identified.

First of all, it seldom pays off to prepare definitions for all items in an instrument. This is especially true for clear and unambiguous items asking for basic information or instructions on filling in the instrument. For example, such items as '*Today's date*' or '*Please check one box for each statement*' are very unlikely to be misinterpreted by a translator.

Besides, providing holistic definitions for an item as a whole is usually more helpful for translators than elaboration of only one, albeit very complicated, concept. For instance, exhaustive background information and a clear explanation of an item '*How much have you been bothered by back pain over the past two weeks*' in the context of the instrument will be of much more value for translators than providing a definition of the term '*bother*' alone. However, this doesn't mean that there shouldn't be definitions of individual concepts, especially when an item or a response option is actually comprised of only one word or a short phrase, such as '*severe*' or '*superficial pain*'.

Special attention needs to be paid to compound nouns, i.e. a group of words made up of two or more nouns and/or other parts of speech. Their meaning may be ambiguous as it is not always immediately clear which word modifies (gives the property to) which word. For example, an instrument title 'General Behavior Inventory' may be interpreted as 'a general inventory of behaviour' and 'an inventory of general behaviour'. Instrument developers will not see any ambiguity here as they know precisely what they wanted to say, but translators, who do not have the same educational and professional background as developers, may have problems with understanding this title. Therefore, compounds should always be explained in concept elaboration.

Moreover, specialist medical terms in most cases do not require any concept elaboration. Initially this may sound counterintuitive, but in fact specialist vocabulary tends to be much less ambiguous than concepts referring to emotions or mental states, which are abundant in clinical research survey instruments. Therefore, it would be superfluous to provide definitions for such terms as '*stethoscope*', '*peak flow meter*', '*dialysis*', as direct equivalents for these words can be found in most languages. This, however, does not apply to the names of healthcare institution and healthcare providers, as these terms vary greatly among countries and languages (e.g. the concept of '*family physician*' has no correspondences in many countries and has to be translated descriptively, depending on the context, so a concept elaboration for this term would be extremely helpful).

Finally, items that need to be explained in the concept elaboration may be identified with the help of translatability assessment (please see section "Translatability assessment").

Preparing draft definitions

Concept elaboration is a means of facilitating the understanding of the source instrument, and not making it even more challenging. Therefore, item definitions have to be clear and unambiguous. Below follows a list of guidelines that may help ensure this.

- Avoid circular definitions, i.e. do not define concepts in terms of other concepts that haven't been defined. For example, a response option *listless* should not be explained as *lacking energy*. Instead, a descriptive definition has to be used which is relevant to the condition that the instrument is devoted to, such as '*A listless patient does not have energy to do things (this is evident in his or her level of activity or through self-report). A listless patient does not show enthusiasm about the things that he or she is usually enthusiastic about, for example, refuses to engage in his or her favourite activity for no apparent reason*'. Even if there is no direct equivalent for '*listless*' in a given target language, with such concept elaboration a translator will be able to find the closest equivalent or render this term descriptively. Similarly, '*anxious*' should not be explained as '*worried*' or '*nervous*'. A descriptive definition for '*anxious*' could be '*a feeling that you get when you are expecting something to happen and you are not certain about the outcome*'.
- Avoid providing dictionary definitions. For example, do not explain '*discomfort*' as '*a feeling of being uncomfortable physically or mentally, or something that causes this*[10]' as

[10] Definition from Cambridge Dictionary (http://dictionary.cambridge.org/dictionary/english/discomfort, accessed on July 7, 2016)

translators can easily look up the same definition in dictionaries. Instead, try to adapt the definition of a given term for the context of the instrument where it is used, or, more preferably, explain the phrase where it is used as a whole.

- Define concepts only in the context of the instrument where they are used. For instance, a tem '*subject*' could mean '*a participant of a clinical trial*' or simply '*a patient with reference to whom a physician fills in a given instrument*'. Depending on the context, this term may have to be translated differently in other languages.
- If a concept elaboration contains additional instructions for translators, make sure that the instructions are not based on some linguistic features unique to the English language. For example, a concept *overall* in a phrase '*How satisfied are you overall…*' was explained as '*taking everything into account*', followed by an instruction '*If possible do not write 'generally' as this is a little different.*' There are languages where this distinction does not hold, so the instruction is irrelevant. The same applies to instructions on ensuring consistency in response options: in English, the adverb *extremely* can be used both with positive and negative features (e.g. *extremely satisfied, extremely dissatisfied*), whereas in other languages different intensifiers must be used (an approximate back-translation from Ukrainian, for example, is *completely satisfied vs. absolutely dissatisfied*). If a translator yields to the requirement and follows such instructions the resulting translation may be stylistically or grammatically unacceptable.
- Offer alternatives and possible solutions based on the experience of translating a given term during the previous projects. For instance, the terms *pain* and *ache* are not differentiated in many languages. If it is absolutely critical for the instrument to have both terms reflected in the translation, then a common solution can be suggested, explaining *pain* as 'sharp, short-lasting pain' and *ache* as '*dull, prolonged pain*'

After the draft definitions have been prepared they may need to be updated based on the results of the translatability assessment process (described below). The final step in concept elaboration is verification of item definitions by instrument developers.

TRANSLATABILITY ASSESSMENT

Translatability assessment (TA) is the preventive medicine of translation. This metaphoric definition renders the exact purpose of TA – prevent translation problems and errors before the actual translation process begins. Such predictive properties of TA have been convincingly shown in a retrospective study [Conway, 2014], where translatability assessment singled out those items that previously demonstrated poor content validity or poor measurement performance. However, there is still no agreement on such basic aspects of TA as the number of linguists to be involved or the number of languages they should represent. Therefore, the following discussion will be based on the scarce research data available and, more heavily, on our actual experience in this area. The TA can be divided into the following steps:

- Selection of linguistic consultants;
- Carrying out the TA and analyzing the results;
- Modifying the concept elaboration based on TA results.

TA can also be used in instrument development (simultaneous development), but this aspect will not be discussed here.

Selection of linguistic consultants

Linguistic consultants that carry out TA should be professional translators with extensive experience in translating clinical research survey instruments. We believe that there should be at least two linguists representing every language that was selected for the TA process. If we invite only one linguist per language there is always a possibility that their comments will reflect their personal preferences and not the actual constraints of a given language.

The choice of languages depends on the needs of the translation project. If the client knows in advance which languages the instrument will have to be translated into, then the languages for the TA will be selected only from this group. We suggest working with a maximum of four languages. This will ensure manageability of data and optimize the comparison of identified issues between the languages. If it is not known which target languages will be involved in the translation process, the languages for the TA should be selected based on the language typology and genetic classification. This will ensure a variety of languages, thus making the TA more generalizable. Table IV presents a distribution of the world's languages along the criteria of typology and genetic classification that will be helpful in selecting the languages for TA. The table uses a simplified classification adapted for practical purposes and lists only the languages that are most commonly used in translation for clinical research purposes. An additional criterion of selecting languages for TA is the graphic system that they use.

	Indo-European	**Altaic, Sino-Tibetan**	**Hamitic-Semitic**	**Uralic, Japonic**
Isolating		Chinese		
Agglutinating		Turkish		Hungarian Finnish Japanese
Flectional	Slavic languages Romance languages		Arabic Hebrew	Estonian

Table IV. *Language typology and genetic classification*

Organizing the translatability assessment process and updating concept elaboration

The project manager responsible for TA prepares a review grid, which includes the original instrument item, its concept elaboration, and place for comments. The linguistic consultants (8 in total, 2 per language) are instructed to review the original items and identify those that will be challenging to translate into their target language. The consultants can be prompted to classify the reasons for difficulties into the following categories:

- Grammatical;
- Lexical;
- Extra-linguistic.

Grammatical difficulties are caused by different ways of structuring the language. For example, English instruments commonly use Present Perfect Tense, which is used to describe events that started at some point in the past and continue until the present moment (e.g. '*How have you felt over the past seven days?*' means that today is also included into the recall period). A lot of languages do not have a formal grammatical category to show this distinction and use only past or present tense.

Lexical difficulties stem from differences in the organization of conceptual content by languages. For instance, the English word *day* may refer to an entire 24-hour period from one midnight to the following midnight, to the period when it is not dark outside, or to the period that people spend at work or at school. There are languages that have different words to describe the concepts rendered by the English *day,* and it may be not clear which of them should be used in a given instrument.

Extra-linguistic difficulties refer to features that are not inherent in the language structure, but stem from real-world referents and cultural differences. For example, a demographic information section in an instrument may refer to respondents' race (e.g. African American, Hispanic, American Indian), which is not relevant to the country where the target language is spoken. The same category of difficulties includes different conventions in recording dates, times, titles, as well as differences in educational and healthcare systems.

After the linguistic consultants send back their reviews, the project manager analyzes the comments, initially for each of the four languages individually, and then across all languages. If the same item is reported as difficult to translate by linguists for two or more languages, it may be a signal that the item may cause problems during the actual translation process. However, it could also mean that the item is worded poorly, is ambiguous, or that the concept elaboration is not clear enough. Therefore, the next step would be to improve the concept elaboration and send the problematic item back to the linguists asking them to confirm whether the difficulty is still there. If the problem cannot be resolved by improving the concept elaboration, the developer should be contacted for permission to modify the original item. If the instrument is not open for review, the project manager, together with the linguistic consultants, should try to find solutions to tackling the difficult items (for example, using descriptive translations, adding explanations and possible alternatives). All possible solutions should be recorded in the concept elaboration document to ensure consistency in dealing with problematic items when translating the instrument into different languages. The project manager prepares a final report summarizing the TA process and the identified difficulties and solutions and submits it to the client.

PENDING RESEARCH QUESTIONS FOR THE PREPARATION STEP

While preparing this chapter we analyzed over 100 concept elaboration documents. One of the general conclusions based on this review is that there is a lack of consistency in preparing concept elaborations for a number of key concepts. Although it was mentioned above (see section "Preparing draft definitions") that

Concept elaboration	Problems with the definition
Distressing: causing anxiety/ suffering	Circular definition (a concept defined in terms of another concept that has not been defined)
Distress: serious anguish, serious anxiety	Circular definition
Distress: extreme anxiety, sorrow or pain	Circular definition, inconsistency
Distressed: sad, upset	Circular definition, inconsistency

Table V. *Sample concept elaborations of the term distress and its derivatives*

every item has to be defined depending on the context of individual instruments, we believe that there has to be agreement on the definition of key concepts, such as *treatment satisfaction, side effects*, *caregiver, distress, symptom, quality of life* etc. Table V offers a selection of concept elaborations for the term *distress* and a brief explanation of why the elaboration is problematic.

Another procedural question deals with identifying the best candidate for selecting items that need to be defined in the concept elaboration: is it an experienced project manager and native speaker of English or an experienced translator whose native language is not English? Intuitively it could be argued that a non-native speaker of English is a better fit for this task as they can spot problems that may go unnoticed by an English-speaker, but this needs to be tested empirically. Similarly, although we suggest choosing two linguistic consultants for each of the four languages used in translatability assessment, research still needs to be carried out in order to identify the optimal number of linguists and languages for TA.

Forward translation

Forward translation (FT) is the translation of the instrument from the source language to the target language. The main players involved in the forward translation step are: project manager, key in-country consultant, forward translators, and a client contact person. A project manager is an LSP employee responsible for a given translation project. A key in-country consultant is responsible for the overall translation and cultural adaptation of a given instrument into the target language. It is typically required that a key in-country consultant lives in the target country, is a native speaker of the target language, and is a professional translator with substantial experience of working with clinical research survey instruments translation. Forward translators are professional translators, native speakers of the target language, with experience in translating clinical research survey instruments. A client contact person is a representative of the client who is available for consultations if there are any urgent issues that need to be resolved, for example, if the instrument includes reference to a concept that is a taboo topic in the target culture. Additionally, the instrument developer or their representative can be involved.

There are a number of methods available to organize the forward translation step:

- Translation by one translator (one forward translation);
- Translation by two translators with subsequent reconciliation of two forward translations into one version;
- Translation by a panel of translators and other experts.

ONE FORWARD TRANSLATION

One forward translation is typically carried out by the key in-country consultant. The project manager sends to the translator the forward translation grid (or a CAT translation project package) as well as the necessary supporting documents: concept elaboration (which may be included directly into the FT grid for ease of reference), the original instrument, any legacy translations, as well as reference materials, which may include a list of client-approved terminology for the target language, the translation of the instrument title that was used in the clinical trial protocol, etc.

The forward translator translates the instrument into the target language, ensuring the equivalence of translation and following possible additional project-specific requirements, such as adapting the language of translation to a specific age group. The translator should consult with the project manager in case of any difficulties or doubts and receive the necessary support and guidance.

Lower costs and time efficiency are the evident advantages of employing just one translator for the forward translation step. At the same time, there is a risk that one translator may misinterpret some concepts, whereas with two or more forward translations this risk is minimized.

TWO FORWARD TRANSLATIONS AND RECONCILIATION

There are a number of competing approaches to commissioning two forward translations. According to the PGP, it is preferable that one of the forward translations is carried out by the key in-country consultant, whereas the second one – by an independent forward translator. An alternative approach is to have two translators carry out the forward translations, and then ask the key in-country consultant to produce a combined (reconciled) version that would incorporate the best solutions from the two forward translations.

There has not been an empirical assessment to determine which of the two options is more likely to produce a higher quality translation. However, both on the basis of common sense and practical experience it can be claimed that the second approach is more likely to produce a less biased reconciled translation. If a key in-country consultant is asked to reconcile their translation with another forward translation there is a chance that they will prefer their own version, simply because they feel a 'personal attachment' to their translation. Besides, they may feel reluctant to show preference to another translator's work so that the project manager does not get an impression that the key in-country consultant is less competent in relation to the second translator. However, these are only theoretical statements, which must be verified by research.

The third alternative of producing a reconciled translation is to let all forward translators and the key in-country person openly discuss the forward translations and jointly choose the best options. This can be done during a face-to-face or a telephone meeting or with the help of a video (web) conference. The advantage of this approach is that during a meeting more wording options can be discussed, producing a synergy effect. Besides, the final reconciled translation, as a product of group discussion and compromise, is more likely to be fluent, easy to understand, and not to contain too much of one person's own stylistic preferences. Finally, there is a higher chance that a group of translators working together will be able to identify some misinterpretations of the original. A possible disadvantage (in addition to other disadvantages typical for group work) is that less experienced translators may feel reluctant to disagree with older or more experienced colleagues.

From the project management perspective, the forward translation reconciliation is usually carried out in a separate document in a tabulated format, where both FTs and the reconciled translation are included. The in-country consultant who carries out the reconciliation is usually asked to provide a brief explanation of their choice. In the case of a meeting the in-country investigator takes minutes of the discussion and documents the joint decisions, and then records them in the FT grid.

PANEL TRANSLATION

The panel translation is different from the third alternative described above in that forward translators jointly produce a translation from the very beginning, during a face-to-face meeting or a series thereof. Besides, there are usually more translators involved in a panel, even up to five or seven. Apart from professional translators, a subject matter expert, for example, a clinician, can be invited to participate in the panel. The advantage of this approach (in addition to all the advantages that it shares with the third alternative of producing a reconciled translation) is that translators jointly produce a final (reconciled) version of the forward translation, so there is no need to produce individual forward translations first. Moreover, a larger number of translators helps to bring the risk of misinterpretation to a minimum.

The disadvantages of the panel translation are more of organizational nature. First of all, it is difficult to arrange a meeting where all translators together with a subject matter expert can participate at the same time. Secondly, a panel approach is more challenging to organize when the original instrument is very long, or when there are a number of instruments to be translated, as the panel translation of such instruments would take a significant amount of time. Finally, the costs of arranging a panel translation can be prohibitive.

PENDING RESEARCH QUESTIONS FOR THE FORWARD TRANSLATION STEP

There have been no studies conducted to date that would clearly demonstrate advantages of a specific method of forward translation over the other methods. When it comes to the profile of forward translators, the only agreement is that they have to be native speakers of the target language. However, researchers disagree in such issues as the requirements that forward translators should live in the target country, or that they should have a medical or psychology background. Therefore, more research is needed that would compare different methods of forward translation, as well as the requirements of the qualifications of forward translators.

Back Translation

Back translation (also referred to as backward translation or back-translation) is the translation of a forward translation back into the source language. PGP defines back translation (BT) as a quality control step that helps to ensure the conceptual equivalence of translation and identify possible omissions and mistranslations. For the purposes of this chapter back translation is understood as a cover term that includes back translation proper as well as back translation review and harmonization. The main players in this step are: the project manager, back translators, the key in-country consultant, and a developer or a representative of a developer (during the BT review and harmonization steps).

Generally, it is agreed that back translators should be native speakers of the source language (which in the overwhelming majority of cases is English). From the translation methodology perspective, this requirement is absolutely well-grounded. However, it is extremely difficult to implement it in real life for a very simple reason: there are just too few native speakers of English who are fluent in other languages to the extent that they can perform the role of a professional translator. One of the explanations for that is the lack of university-level training in many of the world's languages in British or American universities. For example, to the best of our knowledge there are currently no programmes offering Ukrainian, a language with over 30 million speakers, in the UK[11]. Therefore, it would be much more realistic to accept that back translators can be native speakers of the target language and

[11] UCL (University College London) is planning to launch a Ukrainian and East European Studies BA programme in September 2017.

at the same time absolutely fluent in the source language. Moreover, the results of dedicated linguistic research of translation into non-native tongues [Pokorn, 2005] demonstrate that translations made by non-native speakers of the target language are not necessarily inferior to those done by native speakers.

BACK TRANSLATION PROCESS

It has to be stated clearly that back translation is not a mirror reflection of the forward translation process as they have very different purposes. The goal of FT is to produce a translation that is conceptually equivalent with the source, respects all grammatical and stylistic norms of the target language, and is easy to understand by the general population, including people with little formal education and poor reading skills. BT, on the other hand, can be viewed as an auxiliary translation whose goal is to help the project manager get some insight into the translated text and identify possible inconsistencies with the source instrument, which may indicate that there is a problem in the translated text (although not every inconsistency means that there is indeed a problem). With this goal in mind it is obvious why PGP recommend a more literal style of BT, which can only be achieved at the expense of stylistic coherence and even grammatical correctness.

Literal BT is certainly helpful for objective items, for example those that contain instructions on filling in an instrument or ask for demographic information. With more subjective items, such as those that ask about respondents' feelings, emotions, and experiences, PGP recommends using a more conceptual BT. This recommendation is well-grounded, but in practice both project managers and back translators may have a problem in identifying which items need a literal BT, and which – a more conceptual one. Therefore, it may be safer to instruct back translators to produce a literal, word-for-word translation, not worrying about the style, and to encourage them to comment on those items where a literal translation does not reflect all aspects of meaning from the target translation.

There is another alternative to literal and conceptual BT which has not been reported in the literature as yet: the use of a so-called interlinear gloss. Interlinear glosses (or interlinear glossed texts) are widely used in linguistics in order to show the inner structure of an utterance in a foreign language to the audience who do not speak this language. The name 'interlinear' means that the gloss is placed between a line in the source language and a line that contains a conceptual translation into the target language, as in the following example of an utterance in Hopi language [Langacker, 2008]:

Pam	tsiro-t	ngu'a
He	*bird-ACC*	*catch*
He caught the bird		

The method could look confusing at first, but translation project managers usually have a linguistic background and should have no problem in understanding interlinear glosses. The advantage of this method is that it is a truly word-for-word translation and gives access not only to the lexical, but also to the grammatical structure of the target language. Since the interlinear gloss on the second line offers literal translation, back translators could provide a more conceptual translation on the third line (this can also be adapted to a grid format, more common in linguistic validation projects, where the forward translation could be placed in the first column, the gloss – in the second column, and the conceptual translation – in the third column).

Another important issue to consider is the number of back translators to be involved in the BT. Guidelines that advocate the use of only one BT commit a basic methodological fallacy, as with such approach there is no control over the quality of BT (unlike forward translation, BT is not subjected to revision, editing, or proofreading of any kind). Since BT itself is used as a translation quality control tool, relying only on one BT for making decisions about the equivalence of forward translation could have severe implications for the quality of the final forward translation. Therefore, we strongly recommend using at least two BTs. In addition, it has to be emphasized that the back translators should have no access to the original instrument.

BACK TRANSLATION REVIEW

According to PGP, back translation review is one of the most important components of the translation and cultural adaptation process as it helps to ensure the conceptual equivalence of translation. During the review, the project manager compares both BTs with the original instrument, and if there are any substantial discrepancies, the project manager describes the nature of their concern in the comments section of the review grid and asks the key in-country consultant to confirm whether any change is needed in the forward translation. The back translation process in general and BT review in particular were analyzed in a dedicated study of back translation [Tyupa, 2013]. Since the original publication is not widely available, we will present here its most important and relevant findings.

The corpus for the study comprised over 50 clinical research survey instruments translated from English into Ukrainian based on the PGP methodology. In total, 1864 items (i.e. segments that the original instruments had been divided into for translation purposes) were analyzed. During the back translation review step project managers made comments on about 40% of these items. As the result of the discussion with the key in-country consultant about 20% of the discussed items were changed (or 7.8% from the total number of items). These results indicate that project managers identified almost every second item in one or both BTs as quite different from the original. It has to be emphasized that the results could be different for other target languages, for example those that are structurally closer to English. Another conclusion is that project managers should plan sufficient time for BT review into the project workflow.

In order to evaluate the effectiveness of BT review, i.e. to what extent it is capable of identifying errors in the forward translation, a study was carried out. Two professional Ukrainian translators were asked to rate the translation of each item as either accurate or inaccurate. In order to ensure a lack of bias, both of them worked independently and were not informed that there was another translator involved in the same study. The next step was to assess the inter-coder[12] agreement, i.e. to what extent the professional translators agreed on the value of the translation. Cohen's kappa coefficient was used for this purpose, as it also takes into account the agreement between the coders occurring by chance. The translators agreed on the value of 1671 items, with the Cohen's kappa coefficient calculated at 0.8959. The strength of agreement (according to [Glynn, 2010]) can be considered as very good.

The 1671 items that the coders agreed upon were then compared with the results of the BT review. The results of the comparison indicated that BT review failed to identify only 19 items out of 1671 (or 1.1%) as containing an error. Therefore, BT in general can be considered a fairly efficient translation quality control tool. However, there was another unexpected result of the study which may change the traditional view on BT. As many as 110 items that were rated by both coders as correct had been changed during the BT review process. A possible explanation of this phenomenon is that the discussion between the project manager and the key in-country consultant during the BT review step helps to clarify additional aspects of meaning of the original items. Therefore, BT is not only a quality control step, but also an important component of the improvement and refinement of the forward translation thanks to better understanding of the

[12] *Coders* here refers to translators who were marking (coding) the translated items as either correct or incorrect.

source items by the forward translator. Indirectly, these results indicate that concept elaborations for items that have been discussed during the BT review process may not be sufficiently clear or exhaustive and need improvement. Besides, there is at least some possibility that forward translators may yield to the project manager's requirements to bring the FT closer to the original, although the translation could already have the necessary level of conceptual equivalence.

Another important aspect that is often omitted in guidelines on BT review is the manner in which discrepancies between the original and the BT are discussed. Back translation is not viewed very favourably amongst translators, and one of the main reasons for this is that professional translators often view back translation as a tool that questions their expertise. What undoubtedly contributes to such a negative attitude is the fact that project managers sometimes assume that a difference between the back translation and the original automatically means that there is an error in the forward translation. A study which was carried out as part of a comprehensive study of back translation [Tyupa, 2013] provides some support of this claim. A group of four project managers who took part in the study independently reviewed two BTs of a questionnaire made up of 23 items. In as many as 22 comments they directly asked the forward translator to explain why an error was made, while errors in FT were in fact not present in all discussed instances. Another possible way of dealing with this negative attitude towards BT on behalf of translators is to let the key in-country consultant analyze the BTs first and identify problematic areas themselves.

Finally, if the BT review identifies an item as a whole or an individual concept that is challenging to translate, a solution should be jointly sought by the project manager and the key in-country person, such as providing an additional explanation or a descriptive translation. The developer should then be contacted to confirm these solutions. However, the possibility of coming across such translation problems will be minimized if the translatability assessment process described in section "Translatability assessment" is properly performed during the preparation step.

HARMONIZATION

Harmonization is the process of looking for and confirming solutions for common translation problems that arise during the BT review step across all the languages that a given clinical research survey instrument is being translated into. The rationale behind this step is to "detect and deal with any translation discrepancies that arise between different language versions, thus ensuring conceptual equivalence between the source and target language versions and between all translations. This provides an additional quality-control step and further ensures that data from global trials can be safely aggregated" [Wild, 2005].

Harmonization can be carried out during a face-to-face, telephone, or virtual harmonization meeting where all key in-country consultants compare their translation solutions to rendering difficult concepts. The discussion is usually based on the back translations of the instrument, and back translators can also be invited to participate in the harmonization meeting. However, the costs of organizing such a meeting, particularly if it is face-to-face, are usually too high, especially when a translation project involves dozens of languages from all corners of the world. Besides, it is virtually impossible to find the time when all the interested parties can attend a harmonization meeting.

Therefore, a more realistic and practical alternative is to integrate harmonization into the BT review process. A project manager identifies items that are problematic across different languages and discusses possible common solutions with the relevant key in-country consultants. As soon as such solutions are found they are communicated to all the key consultants involved. It is also possible that an item is difficult to translate not due to conceptual differences on the level of languages, but because the wording of the item is ambiguous and not clear. In such cases the developer should be contacted for clarification. However, such situations can be avoided if proper concept elaboration definitions have been developed during the preparation step.

PENDING RESEARCH QUESTIONS FOR THE BACK TRANSLATION STEP

Back translation remains one of the most controversial steps in the translation and cultural adaptation process. Therefore, valid empirical research should be carried out in order to identify the value of back translation as a quality control step. In addition, more empirical data is needed about the advantages and disadvantages of different ways of organizing the BT review process. For example, there are still questions as to which approach is more preferable: the one where BTs are first reviewed by the key in-country consultant, or the one where the review is initially done by the project manager. Finally, research into the harmonization process is also needed in order to identify more efficient ways of harmonizing translations across languages.

Cognitive Debriefing

Cognitive debriefing refers to a preliminary testing of a draft version of a translated clinical research survey instrument on a small group of native speakers of the target language. According to PGP, the cognitive debriefing step performs more than one function in the overall translation process: firstly, it helps to identify how comprehensible the translation is to the target population; secondly, it offers the possibility to test alternative versions of translation if no single version could be identified during the BT review step; thirdly, it helps to identify the concepts that may be unclear to the target population; finally, it may point to other issues in the clinical research survey instrument that may be confusing for respondents. The main players in this step are: the project manager, the key in-country consultant, or, alternatively, an independent cognitive debriefing consultant, and interviewees.

RECRUITING THE INTERVIEWEES

The key in-country consultant is usually responsible for recruiting interviewees for cognitive debriefing. As a rule, no more than 5-8 interviewees are recruited per language. Although this is a relatively small number of respondents, it is nevertheless required that they represent a mix of age groups, educational backgrounds, and a relevant mix of males and females. If the tested clinical research survey instrument is a generic measure, for example, relating to general quality of life issues, interviewees are recruited among the lay population. If the instrument is disease-specific, it is usually required that interviewees have the relevant diagnosis. Special requirements may also apply. For example, if the instrument in question is a caregiver-reported outcomes measure, interviewees may be recruited among actual caregivers of patients with the relevant condition. In addition, the incidence of some conditions is higher in certain age groups, so the demographic requirements have to be modified accordingly.

Due to strict regulations on the protection of personal data one of the biggest challenges is actually finding volunteers with certain diseases for cognitive interviews. Depending on the country and population in question, some of the possible solutions are:

- Publish announcements in local printed and/or electronic media;
- Post announcements in local hospitals;
- Contact local patient support groups and volunteer organizations;
- Ask for permission to publish announcements on the pages of relevant groups in social media, such as Facebook.

The time needed to recruit one interviewee may vary from a couple of hours to a couple of days, so this has to be taken into account while planning the project timeline. As a rule, the lower the incidence of disease in the target country, the more time it takes to recruit the interviewees. In some cases, this process can consume even up to one month. In view of this, some LSPs prefer to involve another professional for recruiting respondents and conducting the interviews – a cognitive debriefing consultant. This person does not take part in the forward translation and back translation process and focuses only on interviewee recruitment, cognitive debriefing, and preparing the cognitive debriefing report. For clarity, in this chapter both the key in-country consultant and the cognitive debriefing consultant will be referred to as 'interviewer'.

CONDUCTING THE INTERVIEWS AND PREPARING THE COGNITIVE DEBRIEFING REPORT

Cognitive interviews are usually conducted face-to-face. However, there are alternative approaches of carrying out cognitive debriefing in focus groups, with all respondents taking part in a semi-structured discussion. In exceptional cases the interviews can also be conducted via telephone or video conferences, for example, when conducting a face-to-face interview would put the interviewer at risk (e.g. when the target population are acute tuberculosis patients), or when a condition is so rare that visiting each interviewee would require extensive travel. Here, however, we will focus only on face-to-face interviews.

The time and location is chosen taking into account the preferences of interviewees. The interviewer briefly explains the purpose of the interview. It is essential to ensure that the interviewees understand the following key points:

- Their answers will remain strictly confidential;
- They do not take part in any sort of a clinical study;
- The purpose of the interview is not to collect their answers to a given instrument, but to check how well they understand the wording in their native language.

After the introduction the interviewer asks the interviewee to fill in the instrument, with reference to the interviewee's personal experiences. The interviewer records the time that it takes the interviewee to fill in the instrument. After that each item in the instrument is discussed in detail. Usually, the interviewer reads each item aloud to the interviewee and asks the following key points per item:

- If there are any difficult words of phrases;
- How the interviewee would explain each item in their own words;
- Whether the interviewee would suggest any changes to the wording to make it clearer.

Most guidelines agree that the interviewee's explanation of items in their own words (referred to here as *paraphrases*) is the most important part of the cognitive debriefing. It is believed that the paraphrases of the items will help to provide insight into how the interviewees actually understand the items in the target language and, consequently, if the translation is equivalent to the source instrument.

Whenever possible, interviews should be recorded on a digital voice recorder. However, if interviewees refuse to be recorded, the interviewer should take detailed notes. The transcript of the interviews or the notes are the basis for developing a cognitive debriefing report. The report is normally prepared in a grid format that contains the translated instrument and a summary of interviewees' paraphrases for each item. There are multiple options of preparing the cognitive debriefing report depending on who conducts the interviews: the key in-country person or the cognitive debriefing consultant. For ease of reference these options are presented in Figure 2.

Irrespective of which option of preparing the cognitive debriefing report is chosen, the following step is to identify discrepancies between the way that the interviewees understood the instrument items in the target language and the intended meaning in the source language. If any differences are found, the key in-country consultant should provide a possible explanation for this discrepancy. If the reason lies in a non-equivalent translation, the key in-country consultant is expected to provide an alternative wording that would be closer to the original instrument and provide its back translation. Besides, the alternative wordings suggested by interviewees should also be discussed and either rejected or accepted. In some cases, for example, when cognitive debriefing results indicate that a certain concept is not relevant for the target culture, the client or the developer should be consulted. Whenever possible, new wording should be tested with at least two or three of the interviewees. In such cases telephone interviews rather than face-to-face meetings are more appropriate. As the result of the discussion the pre-final version of the translated instrument is prepared, ready for the following step in the workflow.

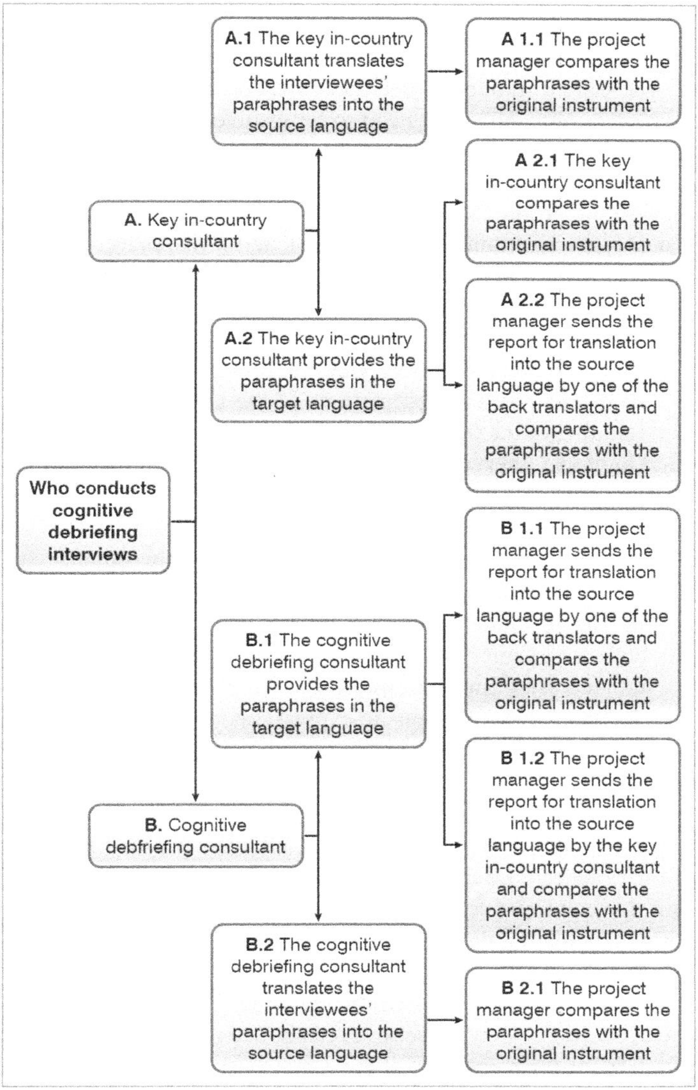

Figure 2. *Preparing the cognitive debriefing report: possible options*

PENDING RESEARCH QUESTIONS FOR THE COGNITIVE DEBRIEFING STEP

There are a number of methodological problems with the cognitive debriefing step that need to be resolved. One of the most controversial issues is, in fact, the basic premise that paraphrases of interviewees accurately reflect the way they understood the target wording. Strictly speaking, a cognitive interview is a variation of a retrospective think-aloud protocol, and it shares its strengths and weaknesses. Some of the most relevant problems are the following (adapted from [Smagorinsky, 1994]):

- The paraphrases of interviewees are themselves subjected to interpretation by the interviewer, so they cannot be considered fully valid representations of the interviewees' understanding of the translated wording;
- Cognitive interviews do not elicit all cognitive processes involved in the understanding of the translated text, and therefore cannot be considered a complete representation of an interviewee's interpretation of the instrument wording;
- The think-aloud model does not take into account additional factors, the most important of which being the linguistic abilities of interviewees (some people simply do not have the necessary linguistic skills to adequately paraphrase their understanding of linguistic expressions).

This means that translation and cultural adaptation specialists should be more critical to the results of the cognitive debriefing, and join efforts in identifying possible ways of improving the cognitive interviewing and reporting process. A broad interdisciplinary research framework needs to be established in order to optimize cognitive debriefing as one of the most critical components in validating the equivalence of translated clinical research survey instruments.

Another problem stems from the organization of the cognitive debriefing review process. As can be seen from Figure 2, only option A 2.1 presupposes that the report is not translated into the source language and is directly compared with the source instrument by the key in-country consultant. In all the remaining options the cognitive debriefing report is first translated into the source language (by the key in-country consultant, the cognitive debriefing consultant, or the back translator) and only then compared with the original instrument by the project manager. The obvious problem with such an approach is that there is no quality control over the translation of the report back into the source language.

A possible solution for this problem would be to introduce an additional quality control step, for example, proofreading of the translated report. However, this would further complicate the already complex translation and cultural adaptation process, not to mention additional time and costs for the client. An alternative would be to let the key in-country consultant compare the interviewees' paraphrases with the original instrument items without translating the report into the source language (option A 2.1 in Figure 2). The key in-country consultant would be expected to translate paraphrases only for those items where a problem was detected, so that the project manager could understand the issues involved. The obvious advantages of such an approach include reducing the time that it takes to complete the report, as well as eliminating problems that could originate from poor translation of the paraphrases into the source language. However, more empirical research is needed into this alternative solution in order to identify its advantages and disadvantages in comparison with the traditional methodology.

Another arguable point in the cognitive debriefing methodology is that it is usually required to debrief all items. This requirement seems hardly relevant to items where interviewees' understanding can be clearly observed by the interviewer, such as questions asking for demographic information or instructions on filling in the instrument. If interviewees are asked to paraphrase all items, this increases their cognitive load, which may reduce their capability for paraphrasing truly complicated items.

A cognitive interview is a form of conversation, therefore, interviewees express their responses through spoken language.

This implies that the cognitive debriefing report cannot possibly capture all aspects of nonverbal communication, which are very important for determining the overall meaning of the message. As a very basic example, there are situations when interviewees say that they understand an expression, but at the same time their facial expression and intonation indicate that they are in doubt. Therefore, interviewers should be specifically instructed to make notes of relevant nonverbal communication into the report, as well as ask additional probing questions to confirm whether interviewees have clearly understood the item.

Overall, interviewees are expected to perform a very complex cognitive task which can be compared to *a vista* translation or consecutive translation. They read a text or listen to the text read to them by the interviewer and then produce a paraphrase in the same language – a process that can be equated with *intra-lingual translation,* first described by Jakobson [Jakobson, 2004]. Such a process puts forward very high requirements to the interviewees' memory span and linguistic abilities: they not only have to switch from a written code to a spoken code of linguistic expression, but also memorize and reproduce fairly extensive excerpts of text. A possible solution would be to ask interviewees to paraphrase the items in writing, eliminating the need for code switching. A pilot study of this approach (Tyupa 2016) demonstrates that it can be a viable alternative to cognitive interviewing, but more research is needed, as with other issues described in this section.

PRACTICAL TIPS FOR THE COGNITIVE DEBRIEFING STEP

The previous section clearly demonstrates that there are a number of methodological problems with the cognitive debriefing step. At the same time cognitive interviewing has been used in translation and cultural adaptation of clinical research survey instruments for almost two decades now. Based on this experience, a number of practical tips and recommendations can be identified that may be helpful for interviewers and project managers.

- If interviews are conducted by the key in-country consultant who also translated the instrument into the target language, it is advisable not to tell the interviewees that the translation was done by the same person conducting the interviews. The rationale behind this recommendation is that interviewees are usually more reluctant to criticize the translation if they know that they are talking to the translator who actually produced the translation. However, if interviewees ask directly who the translator is it would be unethical to conceal it.
- When it comes to checking the understanding of the translated items, it is advisable not to ask a direct question *'Do you understand this item?'* The reason behind this is that interviewees may interpret this question as casting doubt on their cognitive abilities, especially if the relevant item is indeed simple. Instead, it is safer to ask a question like '*Do you think this item would be understood by a person with little or no formal education?'* or a similar question with the same message.
- Interviewees usually have difficulties in paraphrasing translated items, especially when they believe that the wording is clear and straightforward. Instead of asking a direct question '*How do you understand this in your own words*' it may be helpful therefore to elicit the same information indirectly. Some of the possible probes are:
    - *How would you explain this item to a person who didn't understand what it means?*
    - *Can you think of a situation when you felt [acted] that way?*
    - *Can you think of another word or phrase that you would use to describe the same situation?*

Check, Revision, Review and Proofreading

The original PGP devote little attention to the proofreading step of the translation and cultural adaptation process, whereas currently LSPs are beginning to recognize the importance of this step and introduce more and more adaptations and improvements for proofreading. Besides, since most LSPs today work on the basis of international standards, it was decided to build the discussion of this step around the ISO 17100:2015 requirements for translation services. Therefore, such variations of this step as check, revision, review, and proofreading will be discussed below (a cover term *verification* will be used for all these processes). Unless otherwise noted, the discussion is based on the full text of the ISO 17100:2015. The main players involved in this step are the project manager, the key in-country consultant, forward translators, back translators, bilingual editors, monolingual editors, and proofreaders.

DIFFERENT TYPES OF VERIFICATION

Check refers to the self-verification of the target translation by the forward translator. In the context of translation of clinical research survey instruments it is advisable to ensure that translators check the translation throughout the whole translation project. In other words, no individual step for checking is singled out, it should be rather inherent in the workflow as a whole. The key in-country consultant, as well as forward translators involved during the forward translation step and back translators involved during the back translation step, should check the following aspects of translation:

- Completeness of translation (nothing is missed);
- Grammar, spelling, and punctuation (with possible deviations from the linguistic norms in the case of back translation);
- Adherence to project-specific requirements.

Revision is the comparison of the target text with the source text by a translation service provider (TSP) fluent both in the source and in the target language. The primary purposes of revision are to ensure that the content of the translation is equivalent with the content of the source text, and that the translation is suitable for the intended purpose. Another term used for revision is *bilingual editing* (often referred to as simply *editing* in translation workflow), so the TSPs responsible for this step can be referred to as *bilingual editors*.

There is no agreement on when exactly the revision should be done during the translation workflow: before the back translation, before the cognitive debriefing, or after the cognitive debriefing review. Based on practical experience it can be claimed that revision brings the most added value after the forward translation reconciliation and before the back translation. A bilingual editor should be a professional translator with extensive experience in the translation of clinical research survey instruments. The project manager supplies the bilingual editor with the original instrument, the concept elaboration, and any other reference materials that were also available to forward translators. Normally it is required that the bilingual editor introduces the necessary changes directly in the forward translation document (for example, using a track changes function). The key in-country consultant then accepts or rejects the changes. The bilingual editor is then asked to confirm the changes accepted or not accepted by the key in-country consultant. In case of disagreement priority is given to the decisions of the key in-country consultant.

Review, also known as monolingual editing, refers to checking whether the target text is suitable for fulfilling its intended function. This includes checking the terminology as well as the style of translation. In the context of clinical research survey instruments it means that the criteria for selecting monolingual editors depend on the specific type of the document that is being translated. If the document is patient-facing, for example, a PRO questionnaire, it is essential that the translated text is clear, fluent, unambiguous, and easy to follow. Therefore, the best candidate for monolingual review could be a linguist with extensive experience of editing target language texts for publication purposes. If the clinical research survey instrument is specialist-facing, such as clinician-reported outcomes (ClinRO) measure, terminological correctness is more important. Therefore, the monolingual reviewer could be sought among clinicians with experience of working with clinical research survey instruments or technical writers working in the fields related to clinical research. Monolingual reviewers are also expected to make changes directly in the translated document, and the decisions of the key in-country consultant to reject or accept the changes have the priority. It is important to emphasize that monolingual reviewers do not have to compare the translation with the source text, so they do not have to be fluent in the source language. Their linguistic skills in the source language should be sufficient to communicate with the project manager and to provide rationale for their changes.

Proofreading is the final check of the translation. In the context of clinical research survey instruments, proofreading is usually done on the final version of the target document, after the results of the cognitive debriefing review have been implemented. As a rule, no substantial changes are allowed at this stage. Proofreaders have to confirm that:

- All sections of the original document that were intended for translation have been translated;
- There are no spelling or grammar mistakes;
- The formatting of the target document matches the formatting of the source document.

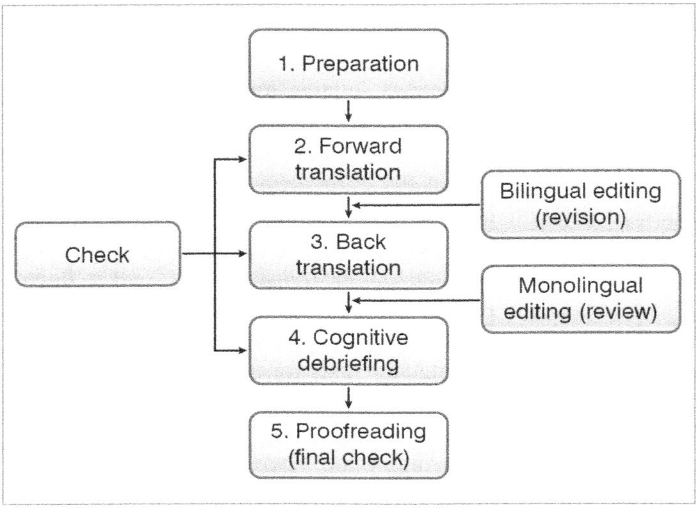

Figure 3. *The place of the check, revision, review and proofreading in the translation workflow*

For ease of reference, Figure 3 represents the place of the check, revision, review and proofreading during all the stages of the translation process.

PENDING RESEARCH QUESTIONS FOR THE VERIFICATION STEP

The division of the initial PGP proofreading step into check, revision, review, and proofreading is a fairly new phenomenon, therefore, there are a number of aspects that require further clarification. The most important tasks include the following:

- Specify guidelines for performing the check step as inherent in all translation activities throughout the project (forward translation, back translation, translation of the cognitive debriefing report, if applicable);

- Identify the optimal time point for performing the bilingual editing;
- Identify the optimal time point for performing the monolingual editing;
- Specify requirements to qualifications of bilingual editors;
- Specify requirements to qualifications of monolingual editors.

Translation of Electronic Versions

Electronic versions of clinical research survey instruments are becoming increasingly popular. They have such obvious advantages as ease of administration, reduced time and costs for collecting and analysing data, higher respondents' compliance with completion requirements, etc. Electronic versions can be developed for various devices, such smartphones, tablets, PCs. An additional type of an electronic version is an Interactive Voice Response System (IVRS), which is based on the completion of an instrument with the help of touchtone telephone keypads. At the same time, the translation of electronic versions has some special features that need to be discussed in greater detail for each of the steps of the translation and cultural adaptation process.

PREPARATION

In the overwhelming majority of cases electronic versions are prepared on the basis of paper versions of clinical research survey instruments. This process is called 'migration'. The modified versions where no significant changes to the content are made are validated through cognitive debriefing and usability testing with 5-10 speakers of the source language [Nixon, 2015]. If the translation of a paper version into a given language is available, then only the updated wording is translated. If there is no legacy translation available, a full translation and cultural adaptation is needed. In addition to the key participants of the preparation step described in Section I, another key person involved here is an IT specialist. An IT specialist is an employee of the company responsible for technical aspects of preparing an electronic version of a clinical research survey instrument. It is essential that the project manager and the IT specialist working on the same project establish successful communication and are available to each other's queries at all times.

Preparation of the source text

The text that will be visible to respondents on the screens of their devices is embedded into a complex programming environment. It is usually the IT specialist's responsibility to extract the text intended for translation into a format compatible with CAT software. Alternatively, the team responsible for migration from the paper version may prepare the text intended for translation before the instrument is sent to IT specialists. In either case, the project manager and the IT specialist should carefully review the source text and identify areas that need particular attention. These include:

- Segments with character limits;
- Segments with interrupted sentence structure (e.g. *Overall, how has your health been [recall period]*);
- Text to appear in pop-up windows;
- Response options.

Special instructions on translating each of these types of segments will have to be prepared depending on the specific requirements of a given instrument.

It is important to stress that translators should be able to modify all segments of the legacy translation, not only those that were updated for the electronic version. The rationale for this is that some segments that were not modified during the migration process in the source language will have to be modified in a target language (e.g. response options). Therefore, the segments with legacy translation should not be locked in a CAT software. However, it should be emphasized that only necessary changes can be made at this point, as legacy translations in most cases are already validated.

Concept elaboration

If a concept elaboration document already exists for the original paper version, it should be used as the basis for preparing

Source wording	If applicable, source wording should be provided both for the paper version and the electronic version so that translators can clearly see what elements have been modified.
Legacy translation (if applicable)	The provision of legacy translation ensures consistency of a new translation with a previously validated version.
Special instructions	Special instructions refer to the following aspects: • Character limit per segment, if applicable; • If a segment has an interrupted sentence structure, then all possible wordings that may appear after the interruption should be provided (e.g. all recall periods); • If a given text appears in a pop-up window, clear exhaustive context should be provided, including reference to the items after which the pop-up appears; • Response options that are identical in the source document may need to be changed in a target language, so response options have to be provided after each item that they refer to.
Concept elaboration	Updated concept elaboration definitions should take into account the new mode of administration of the instrument.
Screenshot	Wherever possible, screenshots of each item should be provided so that translators understand the context correctly. This is especially relevant for instructions that refer to the software options or device options (such as '*next*', '*return to the previous screen*', '*Enter*' etc.).

Table VI. *Concept elaboration document for electronic versions*

a new concept elaboration for the electronic version translation. The primary purpose of the concept elaboration for electronic versions is to ensure that translators clearly understand the place and function of each item in an electronic document. Table VI offers a possible structure of a concept elaboration document with the rationale for each component.

Translatability assessment

Translatability assessment is an important step in the translation of paper instruments. However, translatability assessment is of critical importance when it comes to the translation of electronic versions. It is advisable that translatability assessment is performed as part of any migration from paper to electronic versions, even if clients initially do not plan the translation of the instrument into other languages. This will eliminate the need to make changes to electronic versions after they have been validated.

We recommend carrying out the translatability assessment on the basis of the concept elaboration document template, simply adding another column for translators' comments. As the result of the translatability assessment the following changes may need to be implemented:

- Raise character limits per segment, as in some languages it may be impossible to fit in the required wording under the imposed limitations (e.g. the acronym *ID*, which has only two characters in English, may not be common in other languages. It may be represented as *identification number, identification code,* and can be contracted to a minimum of 4 characters, such as *Id.#, Id. Code* etc.);
- Change the wording of the question stems (e.g. *Have you had this symptom during [recall period]* may need to be changed to *Have you had this symptom [recall period]* as the word *during* may have to take different forms depending on the specific recall period. The same applies to changes

in the grammatical endings in languages that differentiate grammatical genders;
- Introduce additional changes to the architecture of the electronical version. E.g. a pop-up window may need to have a different wording depending on whether the respondent is male or female.

As in the case of paper instrument translation, the concept elaboration is then updated based on the results of translatability assessment. The project manager and the IT specialist jointly work on recommendations of updating the electronic version if the translatability assessment shows that such changes are necessary. The recommendations are then discussed with the client and the developer in order to obtain their approval of the updates.

FORWARD AND BACK TRANSLATION

There are no major differences in performing the forward translation and back translation steps for electronic versions of clinical research survey instruments. Additional improvements include the following:
- At least one of the forward translators should have experience in internationalization and localization, i.e. in translation and adaptation of computer software into different languages taking into account cultural differences and technical requirements of the target country;
- The key in-country consultant should have access to as much of the reference materials as possible, preferably to the original version of the electronic instrument on the relevant device, if it is available, or at least to its prototype or screenshots;
- In order to save time, key in-country consultants should have to opportunity to send their queries directly to the IT specialist.

COGNITIVE DEBRIEFING, USABILITY TESTING, AND VERIFICATION

According to Recommendations of the ISPOR ePRO Good Research Practices Task Force [Coons, 2009], new electronic versions of PRO instruments that have previously been validated cross-culturally should undergo cognitive debriefing and usability testing. As stated in the FDA guidance, usability testing is a "formal evaluation with documentation of respondents' abilities to use the instrument, as well as comprehend, retain, and accurately follow instructions" [FDA, 2009]. Naturally, if the translation of an electronic version is not based on a legacy translation and is fully translated 'from scratch', the same requirement for cognitive debriefing and usability testing applies.

From the translation project perspective, it would be ideal to combine cognitive debriefing with usability testing in target languages. However, in actual translation practice this step is usually limited to cognitive debriefing on the bases of printed screenshots. This is explained by logistical and technical difficulties. Clients may not be willing to send dedicated devices to key in-country consultants just for the purposes of cognitive debriefing. Besides, not all functions of an electronic instrument in the target language may be ready for usability testing, while the text itself may have already been translated. In view of the FDA requirements and the Recommendations of the ISPOR ePRO Task Force every effort should be made to carry out cognitive debriefing simultaneously with usability testing on the type of the device that will actually be used in clinical research.

Relevant modifications are also necessary for the verification step. While check, bilingual editing, and monolingual editing can be performed in a text editor or CAT environment, the proofreading (final check) should be done on a fully functional electronic version of the instrument.

PENDING RESEARCH QUESTIONS

Some of the most important research tasks in relation to the translation and cultural adaptation of electronic versions of clinical research survey instruments are the following:

- Explore whether any modifications are necessary in concept elaboration definitions for items that have not been changed during the migration process but may be interpreted differently by respondents due to a different mode of administration;
- Identify optimal ways for integrating translatability assessment into the migration process from paper to electronic versions;
- Identify and validate specific guidelines for practical aspects of cognitive debriefing and usability testing of electronic instruments.

References

- Conway K, Acquadro C, Patrick DL. Usefulness of translatability assessment: results from a retrospective study. *Qual Life Res* 2014; 23: 1199-210
- Coons S, Gwaltney C, Hays R, et al. Recommendations on Evidence Needed to Support Measurement Equivalence between Electronic and Paper-Based Patient Reported Outcome (PRO) Measures: ISPOR ePRO Good Research Practices Task Force Report. *Value Health* 2009; 12: 419-29
- Croft W, Cruse DA. Cognitive Linguistics. Cambridge: Cambridge University Press, 2004
- Dewaele JM. Emotions in Multiple Languages. London: Palgrave Macmillan, 2010
- Dirven R, Verspoor M (eds.). Cognitive Exploration of Language and Linguistics. Amsterdam: Benjamins, 2004
- Dziwirek K, Lewandowska-Tomaszczyk B. Complex Emotions and Grammatical Mismatches. A Contrastive Corpus-Based Study. Berlin and New-York: Mouton De Gruyter, 2010
- FDA (Food and Drug Administration). Guidance for Industry. Patient Reported Outcome Measures: Use in Medical Product Development to Support Labeling Claims. December, 2009. Available at: http://www.fda.gov/downloads/Drugs/GuidanceComplianceRegulatoryInformation/Guidances/UCM193282.pdf (last accessed July 2016)

- Geeraerts D. Theories of Lexical Semantics. New York: Oxford University Press Inc., 2010
- Glynn D, Fischer K (eds.). Quantitative methods in cognitive semantics: corpus-driven approaches. Berlin and New York: Mouton de Gruyter, 2010
- Harkins J, Wierzbicka A (eds.). Emotions in Crosslinguistic Perspective. Berlin and New-York: Mouton De Gruyter, 2001
- Jakobson R. On linguistic aspects of translation. In Venuti L (ed.). The translation studies reader. Second edition. London & New York: Routledge, 2004; pp. 138-43
- Kornacki P. Concepts of anger in Chinese 2001. In Harkins J, Wierzbicka A (eds.). Emotions in Crosslinguistic Perspective. Berlin and New-York: Mouton De Gruyter, 2001; pp. 255-90
- Kövecses Z. Metaphors of Anger, Pride, and Love. A lexical approach to the structure of concepts. Amsterdam and Philadelphia: John Benjamins, 1986
- Lakoff G, Johnson M. Metaphors we live by. Chicago: University of Chicago Press, 1980
- Lakoff G. Women, Fire, and Dangerous Things. What Categories Reveal about the Mind. Chicago: University of Chicago Press, 1987
- Langacker RW. Cognitive Grammar. A Basic Introduction. New York: Oxford University Press, 2008
- Nixon A, Wild D, Muehlhausen W. Patient Reported Outcomes. An overview. Torino: SEEd, 2015
- Ogden CK, Richards IA. The meaning of meaning: a study of the influence of language upon thought and of the science of symbolism. New York : Harcourt, Brace & World, 1923
- Pokorn NK. Challenging the traditional axioms: translating into a non-mother tongue. (Benjamins translation library, 62). Amsterdam, Philadelphia: John Benjamins, 2005

- Smagorinsky P. Think-Alound Protocol Analysis. Beyond the Black Box. In Smagorinsky P (ed.) Speaking About Writing: Reflections on Research Methodology. Sage Series in Written Communication. 1994; 8
- Tyupa, S. Back-translation: theoretical framework and practical implications. Івано-Франківськ: Вид-во Прикарпатського національного університету ім. В. Стефаника, 2013
- Tyupa S. Cognitive Debriefing of Patient Questionnaires: How to Capture Meaning as Understood by Respondents? in: Thelen M, van Egdom GW, Verbeeck D, et al. (eds). Translation and Meaning. New Series, Vol. 1. Frankfurt am Main: Peter Lang Edition, 2016; pp 283-90
- Wild D, Grove A, Martin M, et al. Principles of good practice for the translation and cultural adaptation process for patient-reported outcomes (PRO) measures: report of the ISPOR task force for translating adaptation. *Value Health* 2005; 2: 94-104

The Authors

Sergiy Tyupa is a professional medical translator with extensive (since 2001) experience in translation and linguistic validation of PRO and QoL measures into Ukrainian and Russian for Ukraine. In 2012, Sergiy defended a PhD thesis on back-translation at the Chair for Translation Studies and Intercultural Communication at Jagiellonian University in Kraków, where he currently holds a position of an Assistant Professor. Sergiy's research interests include translation quality assurance and quality assessment, back translation, cognitive and linguistic aspects of translation, patient interviewing, translation and adaptation of electronic measures.

Diane Wild is a researcher with particular expertise in the translation and linguistic validation of patient reported outcome measures. She has published widely in the areas of patient reported outcomes and linguistic validation. She was the lead author on a translation and linguistic validation best practices paper in 2005 which has become the industry standard for methods in this area. Diane was the founding Director of Oxford Outcomes, a multi-national outcomes research consultancy. Currently Diane is working as an independent patient reported outcome and linguistic validation consultant whilst studying for a MSc in Medical Anthropology

Glossary

BT	Back Translation
CAT	Computer-Aided Translation
ClinRO	Clinician-Reported Outcomes
COA	Clinical Outcomes Assessments
CRO	Contract Research Organization
FDA	Food and Drugs Administration
FT	Forward translation
IVRS	Interactive Voice Response System
LSP	Language Service Provider
PGP	Principles of Good Practice
PRO	Patient-Reported Outcomes
TA	Translatability Assessment
TMs	Translation Memories
TSP	Translation Service Provider

Made in the USA
Monee, IL
04 November 2026

67387163R00049